Intermittent Fasting

Complete Beginners Guide to Fasting: The Science Behind it, How it Works and How to Live an Intermittent Fasting Lifestyle

Intermittent Fasting: Complete Beginners Guide to Fasting: The Science Behind it, How it Works and How to Live an Intermittent Fasting Lifestyle

Table of Contents

Introduction

Knowing what you're doing when it comes to your diet is the most important thing. To accomplish this, you've read articles, watched videos, and picked up books like this one to better inform yourself. However, in most cases, you've been left with more questions than answers as you learn how complex the interaction is between your body and food — not to mention tossing exercise into the mix.

This eBook is going to explain to you, in very digestible detail, what intermittent fasting is and how you can do it. It will detail the types of fasting that are the most popular or work the best and how they do this. You're going to learn about the impacts of food and exercise on fasting, as well as different methods to have a successful fasting cycle. The various methods discussed in this book will teach you how to fast safely, but as with all new changes to your diet or exercise program, you should speak with a doctor or other health care professional before committing yourself to it. They are best able to red-flag any issues that may complicate the process for you, thereby keeping you safe and even providing further guidance for you.

Keep an open mind as you learn the different ways you can encourage your body to change. Try more than one method to see which works best for you — and which, of course, don't! This isn't a competition: this is you bettering yourself. Make each day better than the last and see if your health is improved when you start to fast.

The Science of Fasting

Our bodies are capable of wonderful things. We know, for instance, that when we exercise, we are actually tearing our muscles apart just so they will regrow more densely, thus making us stronger (or faster, or have more endurance). We know that we consume food to fuel and heal us and that if we bring in more fuel than we use, we store some of it away later as fat — yes, that annoying bunch of cells that has made you reconsider diet plans and exercise regimes whenever you see an abundance of them forming.

So, then, where does fasting fit in? We just established that we need fuel to survive. How right you are! However, a short fast is something that can encourage our bodies to be more efficient with how they process food and how they fuel our bodies. "Waste not, want not" as the saying goes.

How Fasting Works

Fasting, as we're discussing it, isn't simply starving yourself. When we discuss fasting, it will only be in terms of fairly short lengths of time without food. Fasting works by depriving your body of fuel for a certain period of time in order to increase stored fat cell usage for energy. The second main concept behind this is that your body will then more quickly and efficiently use whatever nutrients you do provide it with, after this fasting period. Keep in mind that to do this properly, you need to make sound nutritional choices when it comes to refuelling yourself for this to work at its maximum efficiency. This will also instill good habits for you to continue to use when you've finished your fasting cycle, leading to improved general eating habits and health!

Whether you're looking to try a round or two of fasts or implement short-term fasting for the long term (fasts of even as little as 16 hours or skipping one or two complete 24-hour periods within a week), you can expect to see these benefits.

The Science Doesn't Lie

Each year, more studies are conducted to validate (or try to invalidate) the claims that intermittent fasting works. While there are types of fasting that have been proven not to work (such as cleanses), intermittent fasting has some compelling research behind it.

There are a myriad of positive effects that have been credited to intermittent fasting cycles. While each cycle does have a few of its own specific effects, they all tend to have key things in common. For example, in the majority of studies conducted so far, participants became healthier or even lived longer. More research is needed, of course, but what has been done (both short- and long-term) on humans and rodents is largely positive.

Intermittent Fasting Benefits:

- Participants in a study done in 2014 found that, with doing intermittent fasting for 3-24 weeks, they saw an average loss of 3-8% of body weight. These are fantastic results for such a short period of time. On top of that, the weight loss is mostly fat loss — they also lost 4-7% off their waists. The harmful belly fat that accumulates there to create the "tire" that many people wish to get rid of is directly linked to heart disease and other health issues, so this benefit is of particular interest (Berardi; Luca et al 2013).
- Due to the adaptations the body goes through to facilitate a fasting phase, insulin is actually processed more efficiently which increases your insulin resistance. On average, blood sugar was lowered by 3-6% and insulin levels by 21-30% on fasting days. This can even help prevent Type-II Diabetes (Barnosky et al. 2014).
- In general, participants have been shown to increase restrictive eating and decrease emotional eating long-term, courtesy of learning and applying proper fasting rules and strategies.
- Fasting causes your norepinephrine and epinephrine to go up which will mobilize blood sugar when adrenaline is activated, thus creating further fat burn as your body processes and tears down fat cells for their stored energy. Adrenaline release during fasting also ensures

that your metabolic rate stays active and high so you breakdown more triglycerides (fatty tissue).

- Your endocrine system gets a boost — the endocrine system is made up of glands that create the hormones you use to regulate things like metabolism, tissue function, and growth and development. While there are other things the endocrine system is responsible for, those are the key factors that may interest you during your fasting. You will improve all of these areas during the fasting cycle.

- Inflammation sees a decrease throughout the body with fasting. This means that you have less build-up of potentially harmful things like bacteria and viruses in your body that can cause a myriad of issues, and even some diseases. Even looking at the basic, positive effects of decreased joint inflammation from chronic inflammation, you will see greater range of motion and less pain in inflamed areas. That's some fantastic news! On top of that, decreasing inflammation in the brain can have serious implications for further study in areas like Alzheimer's and dementia (Gunnars).

- Your base metabolic rate sees a slight increase and fatty acids are released for energy use. This encourages fat loss throughout the duration of your fasting cycle and will help you on re-feed days when you are eating that ice cream or pizza you've been craving, but couldn't have. Or, when you're doing a regularly timed fast, when you finally do eat after 16 hours or whatever you have chosen, your body will consume that food at lightning speed.

- Human Growth Hormone (HGH) increases. The benefits of this are many, including increased absorption of fats and reparation of tissue. As we age, we produce less and less HGH; fasting is one method we can use to boost our creation of HGH for our long-term health benefits. You will maintain mass and bone density through added HGH, thus off-setting some of the short term losses of muscle that extended fasting can cause.

- Autophagy is increased. This is the body's ability to destroy or purge cells in the body, thereby regulating energy use and keeping cells healthy and strong. When your cells are able to expunge their spent components, they remain flexible and they function better.

Autophagy even reabsorbs the cells that have been tied to Alzheimer's and other neurological disorders. This merits more research because of its potentially life-changing effects for those affected by such conditions.

Intermittent Fasting Drawbacks:

- For this to work, you have to be married to it. The whole point is consistency. Unfortunately, keeping your body in a fasted state requires you to be committed to maintaining your eating routine — no matter what. So, if you are unable to adhere to it, don't start it. When you are able to, it will be the best try you can possibly give it.
- If you enjoy doing long endurance activities such as multi-day hikes, marathons, or other all-day activities, you will need to work around your fasting routine or take a break from it. These activities require consistent fuel, often in carbohydrate form, if you are going to give peak performance without losing muscle (or worse).
- There are times you are going to have to say no to social situations that interfere with your present fast. Mutli-day holidays can be particularly challenging where there are many large gatherings in close succession — you are likely going to see less results during these timeframes; however, fasting can help you make better choices overall and hopefully stave off the worst gains.
- You may miss the meals you're cutting out. Are you fasting during the day? You may miss breakfast. At night? Well, you may miss that supper.
- You may initially notice some mood swings as your body adjusts to the new feeding cycle. We all know that when we're "hangry" we may say things or act in a way that we don't really mean, but can't really help since our fuse is shorter due to hunger. Hopefully this stabilizes for you quickly (within the first week or two), but if it doesn't, perhaps fasting isn't for you.
- You may find that you are mentally foggy or slow until your body adapts, as well. You've become accustomed to the way you eat, so your body expects nutrients at certain times and has actually adapted how it signals you (uses hormones) based around your eating patterns. When there's a drastic change, your body is going

to tell you that it is unhappy, stressed, and worried; once you've gone through the worst of this and your body does what it does best — adapts — you should notice you're back to your normal self, and possibly even feel better than before! But the first two weeks or so can be a challenge.

As always, the more research you do, the better. Look for credible sources that show you what studies have been done that are unbiased and fair. The bibliography section of this eBook is a good start for your own research (look at the studies and the case studies, as well as the personal experiments) and decide for yourself which approach may be best for you. Keep abreast of the information so you can incorporate new trends and research as it becomes available to you. The more informed you are, the better your chances of success will be!

Why it's Good for You

There are many positive benefits associated with intermittent fasting. The most obvious ones include giving a boost to your metabolism through deprivation — remember, intermittent fasting encourages our bodies to be more efficient with how they process food when we re-introduce it — and achieving body-change goals. Whether you're looking to lose weight or increase lean muscle mass, fasting can be your friend.

On top of the list of positives mentioned above, you also can consider the benefits of instilling a more manageable form of dieting into your life. This plan doesn't require you to cut out all the foods you love to eat, but it encourages you to consider when you have them. In general, this helps you because you can learn long-term control from this tactic to maintain food choice control. Following this, you will learn the true difference between real and mental hunger — something we all need to be reminded of, from time to time. Long-term, this means recognizing when you're eating out of some other need than hunger, thereby giving you the leg-up you need to combat these cravings.

Less conclusive research suggests that fasting can lengthen your life by reducing the chance of life-threatening diseases (predominantly of the heart and blood) and even reduce the risk of cancer (possibly due to less digestive stress). Thomas Seyfried focuses research in the area of cancer and fasting to see if extended fasting (as discussed above) does indeed have positive effects on preventing or eliminating cancer cells in the body. This has to do with your mitochondria remaining healthy and entering ketosis, though by no means is this eBook saying that a fast can cure cancer — only that there is research showing this may indeed be a causal factor and another method by which to fight this awful disease. Not to mention, another potentially amazing positive benefit to fasting.

As with any new form of diet restriction, more research is necessary. Only in the last 5-10 years has true, unbiased research really been started on intermittent fasting, so you can look forward to lots of new information coming out over the next few years.

Who Can Benefit from Fasting — and Who Won't

As with all forms of diet or exercise change, there is no "one size fits all" approach. Nothing works the same for everyone! So, while there are many people who will benefit from intermittent fasting, not everyone will. Try out the different methods that we will be going through in the next section and figure out which works best for you. Generally speaking, however, intermittent fasting works for the following groups of people:

- Those who are looking to shed some added weight. This type of diet works extremely well for those who want to challenge their metabolism for change and are already fairly fit. They are used to changing and adapting their food intake to match their exercise needs and their body composition goals. The fast is less of a shock for these type of people because they already know what it is like to eliminate certain foods, restrict eating patterns, or eat for the purpose of refuelling and nutrient intake.
- You want to kick-start your weight loss. Some strategies will need to be worked out if you are looking for a drastic measure to start losing

that weight you've wanted to for a while. Your body is happy at the weight it's at (homeostasis) and will be unwilling to change. You are going to notice many of the negative side-effects of fasting such as the mood swings, etc. a little more acutely than those who have had practice with them before. That's okay! Be mindful and perhaps look into some self-calming techniques to aid you in your transition.

- Anyone looking to increase their lean muscle mass. This style of eating really encourages metabolic success through nutrient absorption and fat burn, so as long as you are comfortable with supplementing BCAAs (as discussed), then you should be fine with fasting to increase your lean muscle tissue. The important thing here is to keep your body fuelled after your workout, so ensure you're working out before your first meal of the day — and make this meal jam-packed full of the nutrients required for success. This will help your body to use the fat stores for energy and allow you to build muscle.

- Those who want better self-control over their eating habits and food cravings. This isn't referring to those who have eating disorders. This is for the average person who wants to eat better daily for their own personal benefits. Intermittent fasting can help an individual learn the difference between mental and physical hunger, and therefore increase healthy eating habits for the future.

And intermittent fasting might not work for these types of people:

- Are you a child? No? Good, then you can consider trying fasting. But, if you have kids, don't force them to fast — they're in a constant state of growth and need that food! Once you're an adult, this is not a problem; but during those crucial growth and development years, don't even think about it.

- If you are underweight, or have a history of eating disorders, you definitely want to connect with your health practitioner before you start this kind of eating plan. The worst thing that you could do would be to feed into your eating disorders by forcing another diet on yourself.

- Similarly, if you are diabetic or take prescribed medications that could be influenced by a change in your diet, you should consult your doctor before starting any intermittent fasting. No weight loss or mass gain is worth your health.
- Some studies conducted on rodents suggested that women could have less control over their blood sugar during a fast, thus having greater difficulties regulating their energy or moods. Some may even stop having their cycle completely — while this may not sound like such a bad thing on paper, it is something to consider discussing with your doctor if it happens. Being prepared is the best way to avoid any nasty, unforeseen complications.
- Also as a woman, if you are considering conceiving, are already pregnant, or breast feeding, you should think about holding off on any dietary changes. At the very least, you should talk to your doctor to make sure it is safe for you.
- You should also reconsider trying intermittent fasting if you have a history of known nutrient deficiencies such as low iron, B12, or vitamin D. Fasting can have a negative impact on these pre-existing conditions, so consider your health carefully before deciding.
- If you have low blood pressure or generally have difficulty controlling your blood sugars, you may not want to give this diet a go. If you decide to, be aware of any changes in condition and consult your physician. Passing out is not an ideal addition to your workout or your day, in general.

Do you fit into either of these categories? Even if you aren't sure intermittent fasting is for you, you can still learn a thing or two about food timing from this eBook — no worries! There are a lot of benefits to be taken away from the fasting concepts, from recognizing true hunger to choosing nutritious foods. So, since you've already mastered the science behind why intermittent fasting works, why not apply what you've learned here to some of the ways people practice fasting.

The History of Fasting

As I'm sure you're well aware, fasting has been and continues to be a part of our world. From various religious fasts still observed today (Ramadan and Yom Kippur, for example) to starvation protests, we see the ways in which depriving the body of food can be used. While starvation protests don't exactly lead to healthier bodies, in most cases, they do make a dramatic point about the greater needs of a person or a group of people that can't be met through food.

Religions have used fasting as a way to clear the mind, purify the body, and help the soul reach out to the preferred greater power. This in itself is interesting when we look at the scientific benefits of fasting — Buddhist monks, for example, are renowned for their amazing and almost supernatural abilities. The monks employ fasting as a regular part of their lives as a method to practice self-control. If this concept interests you, do some research into various religious fasting practices to see what use they are put to and how science currently proves or disproves those theories.

Secularly, we can see a history of fasting in the way in which humans survived. In ancient times, we were hunters and gatherers and therefore most of our meals were not guaranteed or expected. We searched for food, and when we found none, we starved. Our bodies, genetically then, are conditioned to go without food for a long period of time and then potentially feast after. This is why scientists suppose that our bodies have increased reaction and sensitivity to food after a fasting period — it's not just because our bodies need fuel, now! It's also because we need be able to work harder to find that food. We need to be able to act quicker and think clearer in order to survive. Thus, our bodies adapt and provide us with the ability to do so through improved norepinephrine and epinephrine production — when fasting, we adapt to increase our adrenaline output in order to be more efficient hunter-gatherers. Now that's food for thought!

So, if we are conditioned to fast already, why isn't it easier? We have worked very hard as a species to ensure our hunting and gathering limits are within 100m of our homes. Most of us no longer have to work very hard for our sustenance. On top of that, most people don't willingly put themselves into uncomfortable situations like fasting. However, perhaps this is also adding to the obesity epidemic we see in the modern world where there is no lack of or struggle for food. With that in mind, perhaps going back to our roots and re-introducing some level of fasting is beneficial to us for our bodies and for our minds. Keep a journal of your progress as you fast and note your mental clarity each day of your fasts — what improvements do you see over time, if any?

While fasting in the health and wellness world for weight loss is fairly new to the scene, despite ages of history of fasting, we can still see back about 80 years to when fasting for health improvement started emerging. There have been various champions for the fasting movement recently, such as Martin Berkhan in about 2010 when he created Leangains (a style of intermittent fasting) and Brad Pilon who created Eat-Stop-Eat (a type of alternate day fasting) around the same time. This is an exciting time for dietary science because we can finally study the effects of all types of fasting on the body and see if any of our history of fasting can be rationalized with science, and to what extent.

Various Types of Fasting

While there are a variety of ways to fast, you are going to learn about the over-arching umbrella called Intermittent Fasting and some of the variations found under it. The most popular types of intermittent fasting are: intermittent fasting itself, alternate day fasting, 5:2, and extended fasting. Each has its own specific requirements, based off of scientific evidence, as well as its own benefits.

Intermittent Fasting

This style of fasting, in its particulars, involves abstaining from food for a period of many hours. The timeframes most tested at the moment are 16 and 20 hour breaks from food followed by 8 or 4 hours of a re-feed period. We'll refer to them as 16/8 and 20/4 here.

Females who chose to follow this style of fasting may want to fast for only 14 or 15 hours at a time. Their bodies seem to be better adapted to that style of fasting than the 16 hours, but again listen to your body. If you are seeing better results off of 16 hours of fasting, do that; if you find it is off of 14, do that. You can start by using 14/10 and then trying 16/8 to test which is better for you.

This fast may be the easiest for you to enter into in the beginning — think about those times you have forgotten to eat because you were occupied with other things. Did you miss food? You didn't find yourself truly hungry until your body reminded you that eating is important. That likely was at about the 16 hour mark. This comments back to the idea of mental versus physical hunger. We are established eaters. We try to eat at least 3-4 times per day (does "three square meals" sound familiar?) and that breakfast is the most important meal of the day. True! But let's think of breakfast as it is truly meant: breaking the fast.

With intermittent fasting, you are going to fast for 16-20 hours of time and then break that fast with your first big meal — ideally after your workout.

This is indeed the most important meal of your day, so choose what you eat wisely. Decide on foods that are going to provide the most amount of nutrient bang for your buck post-workout. Lean protein sources (meats or legumes, whatever your dietary needs and preferences allow), quality carbohydrates, and minerals/vitamins in whatever capacity you desire.

Frequently, you will see these diet plans with limited carbohydrates involved. This can be either positive or negative, depending on your timing and loading principles. This is a little more in-depth than this eBook is going to get into, so to keep it simple, let's look at using carbs in a positive way with your workout. If you are nervous about consuming too many carbs, then make sure you are eating them directly after your workout and then you can limit them for the rest of your feeding cycle that day. Remember, we're happy to include potatoes, legumes, and other starches in the carb family, so your food plan can include those as well for their other vitamin content and still gain some carbohydrates for energy management.

For the everyday person, however, this plan works well — you can eat everything you ate before, but now you only have a limited window in which to do so. This hopefully means you will not be overeating. Please, do *not* stuff your face! You'll feel terrible, and you may even get sick. During your re-feed window (those 8 or 4 hours) you will have 2-3 big meals. If you get full, stop eating! And, of course, once you've passed your window, you are done for the day. Your body will adapt and you will learn to eat the amount you require within that timeframe without either starving yourself or over-indulging.

On that note, it is likely best not to eat only ice cream, chicken wings, and deep fried whatever. You do want to choose foods that are going to help you be the best you. These are the lean meats, well-chosen carbohydrates, monounsaturated fats, and fruits and vegetables we were talking about before.

You will need to be well-hydrated, so ensure you are consuming the recommended 2-3 litres of water per day. Green tea can also be a useful tool for purifying the body, increasing fat metabolism, and giving an energy boost. Start your day off with 4 cups of water and a cup of green tea to give your body the hydration it needs and also to help your belly feel full.

Let's look at doing a fast of 16/8 and what a potential meal plan may involve for one of those days (keeping in mind that males and females will have different requirements, so do your research and modify accordingly, with special consideration to your particular dietary needs):
Fast from 9pm until 1pm the next day. Workout at noon or so and then eat directly after.

> 1pm — breakfast! 2-3 eggs, 2 pieces of bacon, 2 pieces of toast, 1 cup of raspberries, 1 cup of fried potatoes, and ½ cup of yogurt.
> 3:30pm — hungry again? No problem. Make a huge salad with 2-3 cups of mixed greens (spinach, kale, iceberg lettuce, whatever you have on hand), 1-2 chicken breasts, 2 cups of diced veggies, ¼ cup of nuts, ¼ cup of cheese, ¼ cup of blueberries, with a vinaigrette dressing. Want carbs? Add chopped baked potatoes to the salad or eat with your favourite bun.
> 8:30pm — last meal of the day. 8oz steak, 1 cup of rice, 1 cup of asparagus prepared how you like best, ¼ cup each sautéed mushrooms and onions, 1 cup roasted cauliflower, and 1 cup of peas. Dessert: 2 cups of fruit mix with ice cream or yogurt; or some other small sweet treat.

Were you unable to finish your dinner? Try scaling back the amount or the number of meals. Did you get enough to eat? No? Add in a 4th meal. As long as you have finished eating by 9pm and you start only at 1pm, you are fine. You do not have to eat dessert every day, or at the same meal — maybe one of those days you are going out for lunch with friends and want to have a beer? Go for it. We are focused on restricting the when, not the what, when we fast.

*a note on alcohol consumption: if you can abstain from it most days, that is for the best. It slows down your liver function and therefore fat metabolism, so do yourself and your body a favour and try not to imbibe very often (in general, also, but particularly for this fast).

Alternate Day Fasting

This method of fasting requires that you fast for a 24-hour period once or twice a week. It's not recommended to fast more than that, on a regular basis, since it can have negative ramifications for your health. This is, of course, another method of intermittent fasting since you are going to eat — it is just going to be after a longer fast.

During your fasting day, you should consume enough fluids to ensure you are well-hydrated and maintain your energy. This also can help you feel full at times when you are struggling. You should consume the recommended 2-3 litres of water each day, particularly on fasting days. Other fluids you can consume are those without calories, or very low calorie, like coffee or tea. As discussed in the *Intermittent Fasting* section, green tea can be a wonderful aid. Caffeinated beverages can help keep you awake and alert throughout the day and provide a nice change in flavour. It is acceptable to drink calorie-free beverages from other sources, just use your judgement when deciding what you want to put into your body during a fast.

It is recommended that the day you are fasting, you do not workout — use this as your rest day. You're already taxing your body with a fast, particularly in the beginning when your body is not accustomed to it, so don't overdo it. If you want to workout that day, keep it light and short so you reap the full benefits of the fast. That's the main point of doing this, after all!

Your re-feed days are even more important now because you have denied your body nutrient for so long. Your first meal of the day after fasting should be small ... yes, sorry, you read that right: start with a small snack to allow your body to adjust to digesting food again. You do not want to make yourself sick when you do so badly need those calories. Try to eat normally after that — don't over-compensate and binge that day. The better day to have a food free-for-all is the day *before* you fast so that you can use the excess calories in storage. Have the things you love to eat on that day, and eat normally on your other non-fasting days.

A common method of introducing a 24-hr fast is by starting at either first meal or last meal. So, you can do 9am-9am or 8pm-8pm, for example. Do what works best for your mentally and physically. You may need to try this a couple of different ways before you truly know which is best for you.

If you're doing two fast days, you should space them out so you don't feel weak or over-taxed by the fasting. Pick Wednesday and Sunday, or two other similarly spaced days. Then you will follow the same principles you apply to a 24-hr fast: the day before you start your fast, eat to your heart's content; the other days of the week that you are eating, make sure to choose good choices and not go overboard.

This method of fasting may work best for those who don't want to impact their weekly routine too much (and therefore choose Sunday as their one day). Perhaps your family schedule requires that you always eat a family breakfast together on Saturday mornings. Maybe you can only workout in the evening, after work, so you can't make a fasted workout fit your schedule the way intermittent fasting requires. Maybe one hundred other reasons, but the important thing is: only asking for one day of complete fasting works better for you, and you will still see great results.

Alternate day fasting still impacts your health and body the way intermittent fasting does; it's just a different approach. This approach allows your workouts to happen in a fueled state and also is more flexible for people who snowboard all day (therefore cannot commit to an intermittent fasting cycle) or want to go for a weekend backpacking trip. There are activities that require stamina and endurance, and therefore fuel, which a single fasting day can allow for. After your backpacking trip, you can fast on a Wednesday (even if that's not your normal day) and be back on track.

The flexibility is one of the reasons these types of fasts work so well for everyday people who cannot be married to the gym and eat 6 small meals per day. Timing is everything in exercise and diet plans, but fasting can allow you to choose the times in a manner that fits your schedule — no more hassle or stress that you missed a meal or workout.

5:2

A 5:2 workout follows the restrictive calorie needs of a fast, without eliminating food every day. Instead, 5 days of the week you eat normally and 2 days you restrict your calories down to 25% of what you would normally need in a day. This means eating between 500-600 calories in a day, all-told (Varady et al 2013).

This style of fasting may require a little more math on your part because you will have to figure out the caloric count for food you ingest on the two days of limited eating. There are many tools that can help you figure this out (not to mention the suggested calories on food labels), including many that can be found through a quick internet search. This will help keep you focused on finding the right foods to serve your body's needs on the days you are limiting your calorie intake.

Here is an incomplete list of foods in the amount of 100 calories:
- Closed handful of raisins
- 8 dried apricots
- Medium apple
- 4 ½ brazil nuts
- Slice of whole wheat toast with 1 tbsp of peanut butter
- 3 cups of broccoli (that's a win!)
- Approximately 25g of cheddar cheese
- 80 blackberries
- 1/3 cup of chicken
- One medium banana
- Four peaches
- 27 strawberries
- 125g of yogurt

You'll need to find many more combinations that will work for your dietary needs and that can keep you running throughout the day. While you could opt to either eat 5-6 small snacks of 100 calories each, you could also choose to have one meal of the full 500-600 calories. This is completely up to you and how you prefer to eat during a fast day.

On the days you are not fasting, you can eat normally. As with all fasting, beware overeating on the days you are not fasting. What you're looking for is a net calorie deficit throughout the week so that your average calories consumed are lower, without feeling like you are forbidding foods. In a similar vein as alternate day fasting, you can eat a little more on the days before you are limiting your calories.

So when do you include your workout? You can workout on your fasting days, but you will need to have a snack immediately after. You also should tailor your workout so your least intense days are the days you are limiting your calories. Preferably, one of your rest days will be on your limited calorie intake days. The same general rules apply: short, intense workouts so that you are only working out in moderation. Now is not the time for two hour gym sessions, running a marathon, or training in dance for 4 hours a day.

This method of fasting has proven very successful in overweight patients who followed it carefully. During a controlled 12 week study, the group that fasted decreased body weight by more than 5kg (fat mass made up 3.5kg of that, and they lost no muscle), the triglycerides (fats) found in their blood was reduced by 20%, there was an increase in the size of LDL particles (which is beneficial for reducing your risk of heart disease), reduced indicators of inflammation, and decreased resistance to the hormone leptin by 40% (leptin is what makes you feel full, so if you are resistant to its effects, you'll feel hungry more often — thus leading to weight gain through overeating) (Salk 2012).

If you're not sure you want to give up food entirely, this method of fasting may be your best bet. It also could be your introduction to fasting, if you want to do a trial run first.

Extended Fasting

The other, other fasting cycle. This is different from intermittent fasting because you are fasting from 5-10 days at a time, though there is no definite time limit on this (in fact, there's a man who claims to have fasted for 382 days and that he felt great during it (Stewart 1973)!). This is absolutely not for everyone and you need to consult your doctor before trying it. While, yes, there are those — particularly religious practitioners — who do regularly fast in this manner, they have been taught how to do so by those with authority on the matter.

You will have water during these types of fasts and other non-caloric beverages (as discussed prior, things like coffee, tea, etc.). You can indeed workout lightly to moderately during a fast, but you will have to be careful to listen to your body. If you find that you are more tired, moody, or your workouts are suffering, consider easing off from them. If they're an integral part of your fitness regime right now, either modify what you're doing for exercise or modify your diet by using supplements to get you through with the energy and macronutrients you require.

This fast is probably the easiest to explain, though one of the harder ones to start. You will struggle with a lot of the effects of going without food entirely, and need to be very careful when reintroducing yourself to food. So, interestingly, the first and last parts of this fast are the hardest. If you are unsure how you will handle long-term fasting, perhaps start with alternate day fasting so you can gradually increase your comfort with going without food.

The research done on extended fasting, so far, supports it as a way to lose weight (particularly fat) and to achieve a variety of the benefits listed for the other styles of fasts. As previously noted, Thomas Seyfried has noted that extended fasting can lead to reduced chance or occurrences of cancer. To achieve this, you must fast for more than seven days to enter the proper autophagy stage that can help this (according to his research, so far)(Mercola 2016).

The reintroduction of food can be tricky, as you can imagine — too much of anything can make you sick, or feel terrible. So, you'll want to start with small amounts of easily digested foods. Some suggestions include: broth, crackers, or small amounts of fruit and vegetables. Once you're confident your stomach isn't going to pull a fast one on you (pardon the pun), you can have a real meal and get back to a normal eating cycle. You may still prefer to eat in smaller portions due to your stomach and digestion system becoming used to food again. You may even experience loose bowel movements at first as your body adjusts to solids again. Don't panic! Though, if this continues for more than a few days, you may want to talk to your doctor about it.

Once you're back on track with your eating, you can decide if you want to return to a fasting cycle like 16:8 or if you prefer to eat six small meals per day. For the same, obvious reasons stated for the other diet cycles: you do not want to over-indulge with decadent or unhealthy foods when you're off your fast — your body won't respond very well, and you'll likely undo a lot of your hard work!

What to Eat When Fasting

You read that right: you will eat during your fast. This type of fasting doesn't mean you never eat! As you've already learned, your timing for food intake is critical when intermittent fasting. So, what kinds of food should you be ingesting? Let's look at a list of some of the best foods to have during your fast, and even some ways to prepare them.

What Foods Work Best

Protein

Protein comes from plants and animals that have amino acids. You can get your protein from any source you want, whether it is animal or plant, as long as you're getting the right amount. Protein is the most important thing to consume during your fast if you want to maintain your lean muscle mass. During a fast, here are some options that work well:

- Lean meats such as lean beef, chicken, and venison. While there is nothing wrong with choosing fattier meats (pork and lamb, for example), those meats are not as efficient sources during your fast if they're your main source of protein. Mix and match for variety.
- Eggs are a great source of protein and free cholesterol (which your body can use to create more HDL — the good cholesterol). They are quick and convenient to cook up and relatively cheap when compared to other animal protein. They can be cooked in a variety of ways to satisfy your meal prep needs, from a simple morning scramble to hard-boiled for salads or snacks.
- Quinoa and amaranth are some of the best non-animal choices for proteins since they have the highest sources of amino acids found in plants. A combination of the two will provide you with all of the essential amino acids you need to be healthy and strong. They can be eaten raw or cooked and are used in many different recipes: you can use quinoa for oatmeal and amaranth for a side at dinner, if you desire. Adding in some of these sources of protein will vary your

eating habits, even if you're not a vegetarian, and they are a nutritional powerhouse to boot.

- Soy is another source of alternative meat protein. Soy takes on the flavours of whatever you are cooking it with, so if you want to make pho or a curry, tofu can be a relatively cheap addition that will add protein as well to what you're making. Even using it in conjunction with other protein sources can help a little go a long way.

- Nuts and dairy are another source of protein (though they are higher in fat than some of the other choices out there and will need to be consumed in controlled amounts). Nuts can be consumed raw or roasted, by themselves or in other foods like salads, as coating for meats, or in a trail mix. Nuts include a variety of omega-3 fatty acids, fiber, and vitamin E (to name a few) and therefore, while calorically dense, are a great addition in small doses to your diet. Dairy sources such as yogurt, milk, and cheese are full of calcium and vitamin D, to name a few of the important elements you get from dairy. Our body mutated a digestive enzyme for the sole purpose of being able to digest milk after infancy because we identified its utility as a nutrient source.

- Beans and hummus are also sources of protein. Chili is a really filling dish that is often made without meat (although you can feel free to add in beef, sausage, or whatever else you desire) using beans. The texture, flavour, and absorbent qualities of beans make them the perfect addition to soups and rice dishes as protein sources. Hummus, made from chickpeas, is a delicious, garlicy dip that you can pair with your vegetables for both its flavour and its protein. It's a pretty easy way to sneak some more protein into your day — you can even use it as a dip for breads and crackers, as a spread on your sandwich, or on its own.

Variety is key! Try each source independently, or combine it with the others. You may find some new protein sources you truly enjoy that you hadn't thought of before. Having something new to try when fasting can make you look forward to meal prep and meal time. Also, choosing a variety of foods in each category can help you achieve more nutrient satiation from eating because you are exposing yourself to more of them.

Veggies and Fruits

These two are not created equally, but they are created necessarily. You need to eat both vegetables and fruits to maintain a healthy dietary tract, though there are certain ones that will help you more during your fast than others. The vitamins you receive from veggies and fruits are paramount to a healthy body and successful fat loss or muscle gain. Some of your better choices are:

- Cruciferous vegetables such as broccoli, cauliflower, cabbage, bok choy, etc. These vegetables are powerful vegetables that house tons of vitamins and (in broccoli's case) even protein. They are able to be used in a variety of dishes from raw to stir-fries. Cauliflower can even be used as a pizza crust!

- Eggplants, red cabbage, red carrots, beets, purple potatoes, and purple broccoli can add not just a pretty colour to your plate, but also anthocyanins which help protect our cells and heal our body (including decreasing inflammation). They also have tons of vitamins and nutrients that are beneficial for overall health. Any of these vegetables can be used in curries or soups, or any other way that appeals to your pallet.

- Tomatoes are another quick and easy source of nutrients. As well you know, they are loaded with vitamins C and A, potassium, and antioxidants that help with inflammation. Add them to a salad, roast them, or pop them in your mouth raw!

- Peppers (or capsicum, as they are also known)— red, green, yellow, and orange (as well as the hot varieties!) are packed with folate, vitamin C, A, and B-6 as well as antioxidants. They also are very flavourful and can be an easy to consume snack raw (maybe with a little hummus or tzatziki to go with them).

- Berries in general have a ton of vitamin C and antioxidants. Blueberries and raspberries may be some of the easiest ones to add to your food — toss them into a shake, your salad, or your yogurt.

- Bananas have a lot of potassium in them. This makes them perfect for recovery. Plus they're starchy, so they can help with your carb loading. They pair with so many different foods and sources of nutrients that they are pretty easy to get into your day. You can use them as a substitute for a binder in baking, put them on a sandwich, eat them with peanut butter, etc.

The list of fruits and vegetables you can and should be consuming is far too long to list here, but hopefully you have an idea of what you should be including into your diet: a wide variety that includes multiple colours. Think rainbow when you choose your fruits and veggies. Each colour will help you add specific and different nutrients so you're getting the most out of the meals you choose. Even a simple salad can have green, red, purple, orange, and yellow without too much of a stretch — think about what vegetables and fruits you would choose to make this happen.

Fats

Fats are friends! The healthy ones, anyway. We're going to focus more on monounsaturated fats (those are the kind that help destroy the fat cells in your body, as well as a myriad of other positive health benefits). You obviously will want to avoid heavy sources of trans- or saturated fats like those found in deep-fried food. This list will help you pick out the best fats for your fast:

- Unsaturated fats (mono and poly) are the best types of fat to consume. They can help lower your bad cholesterol and even help your body use stored fat cells faster. Monounsaturated fats are found in things like avocados, nuts (like almonds or pecans), seeds (like pumpkin or sesame), and olive and other vegetable oils. Polyunsaturated fats can be found in sunflower or flaxseed oil, walnuts, flax seeds, and fish. Omega-3 fats are a specific sub-type of polyunsaturated fats and have made their way into the health and fitness world in a big way. You can't make them, so you have to consume them — thankfully, the sources already listed include these, so you won't need to supplement unless you want to.
- Saturated fats are solid at room temperature and found in varying quantities in all kinds of meat, dairy, many desserts, as well as some plants such as coconut (including coconut oil). It's in your best interest to limit how much saturated fat you get in your diet — so maybe don't overdoes on the bacon, just yet. Choose your sources

wisely and be aware that you are going to consume some in your diet, and that's okay. It's when you're consuming too much that it becomes a problem.

- Trans fatty acids — these are pretty terrible for you in large quantities. You get them when you heat liquid vegetable oil with hydrogen gas and a catalyst of some sort. This is called hydrogenation ... sound familiar? Yes, you probably have heard of partially hydrogenated vegetable oil or corn syrup. These remain in liquid states and can be reheated without coming apart, which makes them ideal for fast- or deep-frying foods. They are also delicious, a fact that only adds to their danger — we actually want to eat them, and lots of them! Try to avoid these types at all costs. While there are some naturally occurring unsaturated trans fatty acids in nature, by and large we consume them from fast food, baked goods, and other snack foods. They are also found in margarine, which has its own range of complex debate and research surrounding its benefits and harmful effects.

Discuss with your doctor if you are unsure which is better for you (oil, butter, or margarine) if you aren't satisfied after doing your own research. Many diets lean toward less-processed forms of food consumption, so are more likely to suggest either olive oil or butter for cooking purposes.

You need fats to survive. They're good for your blood, brain, and body so it is vital you get enough of them and the right kind. As laid out above, monounsaturated fats are the way to go. They are very good for you, but also calorically dense, so you will need to manage how much of them you consume. Too much of a good thing can still be a bad thing, after all. When you do choose to consume foods with saturated fats, just ensure you're not overwhelming your diet with them. Avoid trans fats whenever possible as they are rather foreign to our bodies when they are artificially produced — and can be highly addictive!

Carbohydrates

Everyone's favourite: carbs! There are many contending ratios of how many carbs to protein to fats you should have in your diet, but suffice it to say: you need carbs, in some form or another, for energy production. That is their job, after all! However, you can choose if you want the majority of your carbs to come from grains, root vegetables, or other fruits and veggies. You might not have expected to see a list of carbs in an eBook about fasting, but again, this is about being healthy and having a very do-able plan. We are not trying to get into ketosis or follow a fad diet; we are working to stimulate our bodies for change. Besides, if the low-carb or no-carb diet was working for your goals, you wouldn't be reading this! Here's a list of helpful carb sources you can use during your fast:

- Grains are one of the more common sources of carbohydrates. These are found in plants and come to us in the form of cereals, rice dishes, breads, etc. You can probably think of at least 15 different types of grains, off-hand. So, to that end, you have a variety to choose from for your carb sources already. While quinoa and amaranth were already mentioned as viable protein sources, never forget they are also grains and include many of the benefits of grains in general such as fiber, trace minerals (iron, zinc, magnesium, etc.), B vitamins, and even antioxidants.
    - Wheat-based grains have received a bad rap in recent years because of the abundance of material and research that seems to show that there is a lot of gluten intolerance in society. However, this research is not concrete and there are many studies debunking this same idea. Celiac is still a fairly rare condition, and while limiting your carbohydrate intake can reduce some bloating and other effects, the question remains if it is the processing of these grains that is the issue, or if it is in fact the grains themselves. Jury is still out, so go by how your body feels — or if you're one of those who are genuinely affected by Celiac disease.
- Root vegetables are an excellent source of carbohydrates and are not often processed. Potatoes are rich in carbohydrates, potassium, and vitamin B-6 … among other things. Potatoes really are quite

good for you and versatile. You can eat them raw (seriously, people do this), pan fry them, bake them, or even deep-fry them. Yams or sweet potatoes are another excellent carb source and nutrient-packed (chock-full of vitamin A and beta-carotene, among other things). Other root vegetables to add to your carbohydrate-rich list include taros, chickpeas, breadfruit, squash, and turnips. You'll figure out more as you experiment with different meal plans.

- A surprising contender in the carbohydrate department are beans. Beans are full of protein, we know, but also carbohydrates. They are fiber rich, inexpensive, and full of magnesium, iron, and other essential vitamins and minerals.

A further note on carbs. They come in basically two forms: simple and complex carbohydrates. You want to aim to consume more complex carbohydrates because they are more slowly digested by the body, which leads to higher nutrient absorption, better absorption overall (less bloating, better bowel movements, etc.), and they make you feel fuller, longer. Simple carbs (like white breads, sugars, and their ilk) are known to increase fat stores in the body and to also be addictive. We love sugar! Between sugar and trans fat, we have quite the battle in the food ring when it comes to maintaining a healthy weight and body composition. Those examples listed above stick to the complex side of the carbohydrate spectrum; however, there are times when you will have simple carbs (just as there are times you will have trans fats) and that is okay. Everything in moderation! Just be aware of when you are consuming these less-desirable foods in order to maintain control of your eating habits.

When choosing your carbohydrates, pick ones that keep you full, longer and which you actually enjoy eating. Have you ever tried breadfruit? It's pretty interesting, has the consistency of bread when it is cooked, and has no gluten. Maybe try that out in a new recipe to entice yourself into a solid eating plan. Carbs are essential for life and energy. It is estimated that 55% of an adult's diet should come from carbohydrates. With that in mind, and the realization that there are carbs in most things we eat, you should be able to make some great choices for yourself based on your goals and desired body composition to keep you fueled and energized during the re-feed segments of your fasts.

What to Expect While Fasting

Just like any other change in your routine, you are going to have to make some compromises during your fast. There are going to be some uncomfortable transitional periods, as well, where you are getting used to your new way of eating. Thankfully, most fasts are short — unless you've chosen the extended fasting option, you can introduce as much or little fasting into your life as you like! So, for those periods of time you are fasting, you should know how your body is likely to respond.

You will still have food cravings! Try your best to ignore them. When you have a craving, make yourself busy and that way you won't think about it as much. In fact, try to time the days you are going to be eating the least with the ones where you will be the busiest for this reason. Don't think of it as "starving yourself" or being deprived, because you know that this is a short-term method for long-term success. You won't be without forever, and you can plan your fasting days around your social schedule so you won't miss Mike's birthday or Jess' going away party.

Your eating cycle will be altered. This is obvious, sure, but keep this in mind during your working day — if you are doing a full-day fast and they surprise you at lunch with something yummy … this is one of those times you will have to make a sacrifice, unless you want to rework your entire fasting cycle. Not only that, but, depending on your schedule (work, kids, sports, etc.), you may need to adjust when you eat. This includes lunch, but also dinner with the family or your last meal after your workout. Expect to become hungry at different times from before, or to feel less hungry overall — this last point is important, because when it comes to refuelling, you need to eat when you're supposed to, even if you're not feeling hungry in that moment. You will need to break that fasting cycle, and while it may sound laughable now, it does happen! You can lose the desire to eat.

Your home time will be different than before. Perhaps you and your significant other used to watch movies and have snacks at 10pm on Fridays. Now that you're doing an intermittent fast, you have decided to be done eating by 8pm *every day*. What to do? Talk to your partner. He or she will understand your goals. If you really treasure those M&Ms on Friday, then maybe consider trying an alternate day fast instead to allow for this activity. Other situations you may run into are changing meal times, surprise treats, or discomfort when consuming certain foods after a fasting period. Your body will process foods a little differently after a fasting period — sometimes this efficiency means that old favourite treats will no longer sit well with your stomach or digestive track. You'll find this all out in time, but don't be caught unawares when you have a strange bowel movement or cramps from a food you no longer consume regularly.

Workouts may be difficult to complete. You'll have to be very diligent when planning when you're going to workout. This follows suit from changing your meal times — you may need to alter when you workout, or be willing to skip a workout entirely. We touched on this briefly in the section about types of fasting. As you can expect, working out during an extended fast can be counterproductive to your fasting goals. You want to keep that mass you've worked so hard to achieve! Your body is more likely to chew up your muscle before it goes after the fat if it feels it needs to repair itself right away. The muscle is far more easily accessible to your hungry body than the fat is, so it won't waste the time trying to metabolise the fat when the muscle is readily available. Can you minimize this? Read on.

What Kind of Exercise Can You Do While Fasting?

You absolutely can — and should — workout while fasting. So what kind of exercise is best? Moderate is the general answer. You want to keep shorter duration workouts so you don't enter into that problem we discussed in *What to Expect While Fasting* where you lose muscle, not just fat. While you will lose some lean mass (likely in the form of water) during a fast, especially at first as your body is adjusting to the new eating routine, you don't want to lose your hard-earned muscle. Fasting puts you in a state where you need to efficiently use your calories during a workout. So, as with most intense workout plans (those in which you use all of your stored energy for powerful lifts, personal bests, etc.), you can choose to supplement with branch chain amino acids during your workouts to help off-set the potential muscle loss.

If you are doing intense workouts, keep them short! The timeframe is what matters, here. You won't be able to do marathons, for example, but you can do short, intense lifts to increase lean mass. If part of what you're looking for with fasting is gaining muscle mass, you are going to have to increase your lean protein intake in order to make this possible — you have a limited window to put calories back into your body, so use it wisely.

Also, in order to maintain better fuel consumption and fat burn, you will need to eat directly after your workouts. Yep, you read that right: you'll eat *after* your workout. So this means you will be doing your workouts in your fasted state. While this works best with intermittent fasting and alternate day, extended fasting isn't geared for doing workouts without losing muscle mass. You can still do some exercise, and you should as it is good for the body, but keep it simple and keep it short. Feeling good during your fast is important!

Some benefits of exercising while fasting are as follows:
- Increased explosive response (short sprints, jumps, etc.).
- Increased blood flow and circulation, combined with your already well-conditioned blood sugar and insulin response, leads to a good pump and better body response to exercise (although, notably, good nutrition and exercise can also create this effect in other combinations).
- Improved fat metabolism and fat loss.
- Improved endocrine system response.
- Increase lean muscle mass.
- Better body composition.

We have overviewed the benefits of fasting on its own earlier in this eBook. Workouts only serve to amplify the effects fasting can have on your body. When timed properly (e.g., when doing a fasted workout), you will see an improvement in the areas you are already targeting in your fasting.

Keep your workouts about 45 minutes long so you aren't over-taxing your body. No one wants regression. As long as you do this, eat well when you end your fast, and hydrate properly, you should have consistent results in your workouts. You should not see a decrease in performance, neither should you feel generally weak or tired during. If you do, you likely need to do one of two things: eat more (if you're doing alternate day fasting, perhaps only do one 24-hr fast) or workout less/less intensely. Monitor yourself and keep tabs with your health care providers (doctors, coaches, etc.) for guidance.

What Kind of Progress Should You See?

As with any new eating or exercise regime, you can expect there will be some fluctuations throughout your week. While overall you can expect to lose 3-8% body weight (and a bit off your waist!) within your first 3-24 weeks, the important thing to remember is that there may be some up and down to start. However, over time, you should expect to see weight loss throughout your fast, no matter which type you've chosen. The weight loss should be steady, and while some fasts may cause you to lose more weight (because some fasts may cause you to lose muscle, as discussed), you should notice these effects no matter which fast you've chosen.

You should see a decrease in fat and an increase in muscle mass (unless you're doing an extended fast) once your body has normalized. Your clothes will fit differently, you will move differently, and your taste in food may even change as your pallet is cleansed through fasting.

After you've been on a fast for about a week or so, you should notice you aren't feeling as hungry as you used to. Your body has adapted to the new eating schedule and you should be able to get through your fasts a little easier. In fact, your body will have stopped craving food at the times it used to be accustomed to being fed at and now will crave food to the new schedule you have forced it into. This is great progress because it shows your body is adapting and it will then be easier on you to continue your fast.

Your mood will stabilize if you're at the right level of fasting for yourself — if it hasn't stabilized after about 10 days, you will need to consider one of the options we discussed earlier: either change your fasting cycle by decreasing your fasting days or decrease your workout intensity.

There's a chance you may have to change what activities you do at what times. Perhaps you aren't focusing as well in the afternoon as you were before. Well, try to move those activities to the morning when you are more critically alert. You should notice increased clarity since you have simplified your eating routine and made the appropriate adjustments to decrease the negative effects of having too much fat on your body (lethargy, trouble focusing, etc.).

How Can You Track Your Progress?

Start by recording your weight before you start your plan, as well as your measurements. Take before photos. This combination is the best way to see your true success from home. If you have a gym membership or access to coaching staff, you can ask them to help you with these things.

Your doctor can also help you with some important measurements like blood pressure, cholesterol levels, blood sugars, and other specific medical testing that cannot be done at home. If this interests you, then try to book in with your doctor about once a month to keep track of these measurements. These can be some of the better measures of your true health because they are internal factors that are directly influenced by diet and exercise, as opposed to strict body image (just because a person is thin, doesn't mean their healthy inside; vice versa for someone who is very muscular).

Pick a day and a time that is consistent, week-to-week, in order to show your true results. As mentioned before, you may notice some fluctuations early on, but this baseline will help you realize the true effects later on. Not only that, but if you see a 1-2 pound fluctuation in a week, that is nothing to be concerned about; in fact, that is quite normal.

As your fast goes on, you will now have a baseline and a consistent measurement schedule to help keep you focused and on track. It is important that you eliminate as many variables as possible so you get the most accurate results possible.

Other, less scientific, ways to measure your progress is to keep track of how you feel each week, both in terms of general feelings about the fasting, but also in regards to how you are feeling on a mental and physical level. Notice how your clothes fit differently as the weeks go by. Do you have a particular pair of pants or a shirt that is a little too tight or ill-fitting right now for you to feel comfortable in? Add it to your assessment each week and see how your body is adapting by how that article of clothing is starting to fit. Maybe you are increasing your muscle size and you have a shirt you need to fill out more — this is the same situation: try it each week to see when it finally looks the way you want to. The pictures help a lot with this because as you go through each week, you can see physical changes you may not notice in the mirror. We look at ourselves a lot during a day, so the captured image of a photo can help us realize the differences when we put them side by side.

Energy levels may also change as you go through the process. They may go up and down as the weeks go on, so keep track of these, too. You may be able to problem solve some issues by reflecting on when you feel tired and how long your bouts of lethargy last. Sometimes caffeine will help you through these times, if you find you're truly struggling, or perhaps even a nap. Napping may help get you through some of your cravings and provide you with a mental boost as well.

Weight Loss Effects

Surprisingly, there are positives and negatives associated with losing weight. We have discussed many of the positives already, but some of the negative side effects can be things like loose skin, seeing stretch marks that you didn't notice before, having to buy all-new clothes (this can be an expensive task!), and having to adjust certain medications that depend on hormone and weight balance.

These negative effects can often be off-set by patience, determination, and your doctor's assistance. Once you've figured out that living a healthy, fit life is well-worth these potential set-backs, you will overcome any obstacles set in your path and embrace the new you.

You will likely have more energy and feel more confidence than you had before. Your workouts will get more complicated and fun, and you'll notice you're capable of more types of activity than before. With some coaching or personal training assistance, or by doing a ton of research and hopefully getting experienced feedback from someone who knows how to workout properly, you will be able to try new exercises in and out of the gym. This will help you overcome any potential stagnation that can happen when your body adjusts and creates a new homeostasis that you need to work past.

When you lose healthy amounts of weight, you become more trim and fit. You may find yourself open to new experiences like ziplining or scuba diving that you didn't feel confident trying before. Perhaps you'll join that sports team you wanted to, but never felt fit enough for. The confidence you will feel by representing your best self, through your hard work and determination will show through when you have adjusted to your own transformation. Wear that outfit, try that activity, be competitive with yourself for your personal best in running or lifting.

Preparing for and Preventing Setbacks

Inevitably, you are going to run into obstacles. Some of them are going to throw you off course — sorry, but it is bound to happen! Life is going on around you, and it could throw you a curveball like an unexpected pregnancy (whether yourself or your partner) or a vacation opportunity that prevents you from eating as you had planned. Even if something like this happens, there are some steps you can do to prepare for and prevent some of these setbacks.

Have a backup plan: you may have your heart set on a specific fasting plan, but keep.a backup ready just in case. If you are getting off track regularly, the plan you've chosen isn't working for you, so try your backup plan! Have your reasons ready for why you can't join in a night of drinking, or have that treat. Your friends and family will respect your decisions, and likely appreciate the head's up that you are fasting! You know, just in case you are moody.

Don't put yourself in situations that you know might tempt you until your fast is over. If you know your best friend's birthday is coming up, but you want to do an extended fast, make sure that you have enough time to do your fast and recover from it before that day. Otherwise, have your backup plan ready to go! Try to minimize that kryptonite food you have lying around the house, even now. Are you a chips person? Or maybe a cookie monster? Make it so you have to consciously plan and act to get these favourite snacks so you are less likely to do so. This will protect your fasting plan and also your waistline.

Plan early and plan often. If you start with a well-rounded plan for your meals and your workouts, you have a better chance of succeeding. Plan them out as far in advance as possible so you don't have to worry about last minute adjustments — or, worse, so you don't get stuck when you lose your motivation to workout or stick to your fasting regime. Whether this entails planning detailed meals each day for your plan, scheduling your workout and fasting times appropriately, or even creating workout programs for yourself for the duration of your fast, you are in control of every step you take. It may help you to plan all these things, or at least sketch them out, so that you don't put yourself in a situation where you have to use your backup plan as your main plan!

Ask for help. Again, tell your family and friends what you are planning to do. If you have a partner, while you shouldn't expect anyone to join you in this endeavour unless he or she wants to, you can ask them to help you through the worst times. Maybe they can do more meal prep so you don't have to work with food if you're struggling with your fast. Perhaps they can plan your re-feed days with an exciting dinner out together to celebrate your success. If all else fails, they're a sympathetic ear when the going gets tough.

Conclusion

Fasting is not for everyone. You may be nodding your head (or cursing under your breath) at this point in agreement. However, it will teach you many things including the limit to which you can push your body and your mind. You are able to try new things, stay focused, and survive short-term fasting. Knowing you don't need food in quite the same way you may have needed it before is liberating. You have the control to back away from the treats, sweets, and deep-fried deliciousness of the world when you need to — that in itself is worthy of congratulations! Impulse control is something many people lack, and it is one of the main causes of self-sabotage.

Fasting can be very beneficial, not only for your physical body but also for your mind. You know the science behind it: fasting helps you lose stomach fat, improve your endocrine system's performance, and potentially even stave off some pretty serious diseases. On top of that, you are gaining control of your mental state and energy levels as you continue to improve your fasting skills. Seeing is believing, so as you continue to record and track your progress, remember to challenge yourself in your workouts and food choices so you continue to make positive changes.

If you've found intermittent fasting works and works well for you, that's great. You now have a new and powerful tool to add to your arsenal to help cultivate the type of body you want, inside and out. It's not easy to change how you eat, but you can see and feel its effectiveness. Congratulations on persevering and accomplishing one of your goals. Now you understand that you are in control of what you put into your body and when, and you are actively able to control this. Apply this to your life in general and you are unstoppable!

As dedicated as you are to your health and wellness, you know above anyone else how your body feels. If you gain nothing else from trying out intermittent fasting, focus on how well your body adapts to new things and how much more in tune you are with your body. You're noticing things you didn't notice before! Apply this to more mindful movements, eating habits, and even lifestyle habits.

Description

You've tried everything to make your body the way you want it to be. You've worked out — hard — and you've followed every diet under the sun. You're frustrated with the lack of progress, the roller coaster of weight loss followed by increased weight gain, and frankly with yourself. You're not alone in this! The good news is: there is a simple format you can follow to give yourself the break you need to have the body you wanted.

Is it easy? Yes and no. It's not harder than anything else you've tried, but it does require consistency. And it works for your everyday life! You don't have to give up the food you love, just the time you choose to eat it at. The chapters in this book will discuss why intermittent fasting works, the tips and strategies you need to effectively do it, and methods to avoid falling off the wagon. This eBook includes:

- Information on what to eat when fasting
- Various styles of fasting and how they're done
- Mastering food content and meal composition
- What kind of workouts can be done by fasting, and when they should be done
- Tips on how to survive your fasting cycles, without feeling like you're starving
- The science behind intermittent fasting
- The results you should see from a fast and how to measure them
- And much more!

Even if you are a pro at the gym and enter fitness competitions, intermittent fasting can give you an edge to cutting down without losing lean muscle mass — without having to go into a carb-restriction cycle. You can share your new eating plan with your gym mates and plan together so you have a sympathetic ear and someone to feast with. This eBook will give you confidence and satisfaction with your fitness life. After all, what's the point of killing yourself in the gym if you're still unhappy with how you feel and look? The last thing you want is to feel like you're wasting your time. So give yourself a little boost and try out intermittent fasting!

Bibliography

Barnosky, A. R.; Hoddy, K. K.; Unterman, T. G.; Varady, K. A. (2014). Intermittent fasting vs daily calorie restriction for type 2 diabetes prevention: A review of human findings. *Translational Research*. 164 (4): 302-11. Retrieved February 11, 2017 from https://www.ncbi.nlm.nih.gov/pubmed/24993615

Berardi, J. All About Intermittent Fasting, in Under 10 Minutes. Precision Nutrition. Retrieved February 13, 2017 from http://www.precisionnutrition.com/intermittent-fasting/summary

Bhutani, S., Klempel, M. C., Kroeger, C. M., Aggour, E., Calvo, Y., Trepanowski, J. F., et al. (2013). Effect of exercising while fasting on eating behaviors and food intake. *Journal of the International Society of Sports Nutrition, 10*(1), 50. Retrieved February 12, 2017 from https://www.ncbi.nlm.nih.gov/pubmed/24176020

Gunnars, K. Intermittent Fasting 101 – The Ultimate Beginner's Guide. *Authority Nutrition*. Retrieved February 11, 2017 from https://authoritynutrition.com/intermittent-fasting-guide/

Klempel, M. C., Kroeger, C. M., & Varady, K. A. (2013). Alternate day fasting (ADF) with a high-fat diet produces similar weight loss and cardio-protection as ADF with a low-fat diet. *Metabolism*, 62(1), 137-143. Retrieved February 12, 2017 from https://www.ncbi.nlm.nih.gov/pubmed/22889512

Luca, F.; Perry, G.H.; & Di Rienzo, A. (2014). Evolutionary Adaptions to Dietary Changes. *Annual Review of Nutrition*. Retrieved February 14, 2017 from https://www.ncbi.nlm.nih.gov/pmc/articles/PMC4163920/

Mercola, J. (2016) Cancer as a Metabolic Disease — A New Look at an Old Foe. *Mercola*. Retrieved February 13, 2017 from http://articles.mercola.com/sites/articles/archive/2016/08/07/cancer-metabolic-disease.aspx

Salk Institute for Biological Studies. (2012). Extended daily fasting overrides harmful effects of a high-fat diet: Study may offer drug-free intervention to prevent obesity and diabetes. *Science Daily*. Retrieved February 12, 2017 from https://www.sciencedaily.com/releases/2012/05/120517131703.htm

Stewart, W.K. & Flemning, L. (1973). Features of a successful therapeutic fast of 382 days' duration. *Postgrad Medical Journal*. Retrieved February 14, 2017 from (https://www.ncbi.nlm.nih.gov/pmc/articles/PMC2495396/

Stipp, D. (2013). How Intermittent Fasting Might Help You Live a Longer Healthier Life. *Scientific American*. Retrieved February 13, 2017 from https://www.scientificamerican.com/article/how-intermittent-fasting-might-help-you-live-longer-healthier-life/

Varady, K.A.; Bhutani S.; Klempel M.C.; Trepanowski J.F.; Haus J.M.; Hoddy K.K.; & Calvo Y. (2013). Alternate day fasting for weight loss in normal weight and overweight subects: a randomized controlled trial. *Medline*. Retrieved February 12, 2017 from https://www.ncbi.nlm.nih.gov/pubmed/24215592 5:2

Zauner, C., Schneeweiss, B., Kranz, A., Madl, C., Ratheiser, K., Kramer, L., ... & Lenz, K. (2000). Resting energy expenditure in short-term starvation is increased as a result of an increase in serum norepinephrine. *The American Journal of Clinical Nutrition*, 71(6), 1511-1515. Retrieved February 13, 2017 from https://www.ncbi.nlm.nih.gov/pubmed/10837292